THE Skinny SLOW COOKER SUMMER RECIPE BOOK

CookNation

The Skinny Slow Cooker Summer Recipe Book
Fresh & Seasonal Summer Recipes For Your Slow
Cooker. All Under 300, 400 & 500 Calories.

A Bell & Mackenzie Publication
First published in 2014 by Bell & Mackenzie Publishing
Limited.
Copyright © Bell & Mackenzie Publishing 2014

ISBN 978-1-909-855-38-0

A CIP catalogue record of this book is available from the
British Library

Disclaimer
The information and advice in this book is intended as
a guide only. If using the recipes as part of a diet, any
individual should independently seek the advice of a
doctor or health professional before embarking on any
diet or weight loss plan. We do not recommend a calorie
controlled diet if you are pregnant, breastfeeding, elderly
or under 18 years of age. Some recipes may contain nuts or
traces of nuts. Those suffering from any allergies associated
with nuts should avoid any recipes containing nuts or nut
based oils.

Contents

Contents

Contents

Introduction

It's time to get creative with your slow cooker this summer. If you think the slow cooker is only good for hearty, soul warming soups and stews in the colder months, then it's time to open your mind and your kitchen to a whole new world of summer possibilities.

Yes it's true that many of us only let our slow cookers see the light of the day when the nights begin to draw in and the temperature drops, but really there is absolutely no reason why you shouldn't make use of this amazingly versatile appliance all year round. There are so many dishes that can be cooked in the slow cooker and they can be just as light and refreshing as any cooked in an oven or stove-top. From skinny summer suppers that highlight the flavours of the season to smoky barbeque cuts...you name it, the slow cooker cooks it!

We already know that the slow cooker is an extremely economical as well as convenient method of cooking. In the summer months when the temperature rises, using a conventional oven turns up the heat in your kitchen and can make it uncomfortable. The slow cooker doesn't emit much heat beyond the pot so it helps keep you and your kitchen cooler. What's more it uses far less energy than a conventional oven so you're saving energy too.

One of the best things about slow cooker cooking is that it takes care of itself leaving you to attend to other things. What better appliance to have in the kitchen in the beautiful summer months? The slow cooker can be your new best friend allowing you to enjoy the weather, friends and family while the slow cooker does all the work.

Our skinny collection of summer recipes are perfect for those wishing to maintain a balanced, healthy diet. Each recipe serves four people and all fall below either 300, 400 or 500 calories. We have tried to make the best of seasonal fresh ingredients, although of course there are some staples which are not just summer fare and store cupboard items which you'll use all year round . If you are following a calorie-controlled diet these delicious slow cooking summer recipes can be the perfect companion to keep your weight loss efforts on track while still making the best of the summer.

So it's time to put away your preconceptions and open up to a world of seasonal, fresh, light and healthy summer slow cooker recipes...all under 300, 400 and 500 calories.

The slow cooker is this summer's 'must-have' kitchen appliance!

The Skinny Slow Cooker Summer Recipe Book compliments the hugely successful range of skinny slow cooker titles by CookNation. You may also enjoy....

- *The Skinny Slow Cooker Recipe Book*
  #1 Amazon Best Seller
- *More Skinny Slow Cooker Recipes*
- *The Skinny Slow Cooker Vegetarian Recipe Book*

- *The Skinny Slow Cooker Soup Recipe Book*
- *The Skinny Slow Cooker Curry Recipe Book*
  #1 Amazon Best Seller
- *The Skinny 5:2 Diet Slow Cooker Recipe Book*
  #1 Amazon Best Seller
- *The Paleo Diet For Beginners Slow Cooker Recipe Book*

If you have already read one of the other 'Skinny' titles from CookNation you may be familiar with some of the following information, in which case please feel free to skip straight to our recipes. If however your slow cooker has been stored in a cupboard or you have just purchased a slow cooker for the first time, we recommend reading the following pages to familiarise yourself with how to get the best out of your appliance and advice on using our recipes.

Cooking The Skinny Way
Many of us can be guilty of overeating and making poor nutritional choices, which can often result in overeating, weight gain and sluggishness.

These delicious summer slow cooker recipes use simple, seasonal and inexpensive fresh and store-cupboard ingredients, are packed full of flavour and goodness, and show that you can enjoy maximum taste with minimum calories.

Each recipe has been tried, tested, and enjoyed time and time again and we're sure you'll soon agree that diet can still mean delicious!

Preparation

Most of the recipes should take no longer than 10-15 minutes to prepare. Browning the meat will make a difference to the taste of your recipe, but if you really don't have the time, don't worry - it will still taste great.

All meat and vegetables should be cut into even sized pieces unless stated in the recipe. Some ingredients can take longer to cook than others, particularly root vegetables, but that has been allowed for in the cooking time.

As much as possible meat should be trimmed of visible fat and the skin removed.

Low Cost

Slow cooking is ideal for cheaper meat cuts. The 'tougher' cuts used in this collection of recipes are transformed into meat which melts-in-your-mouth and helps to keep costs down. We've also made sure not to include one-off ingredients, which are used for a single recipe and never used again. All the herbs and spices listed can be used in multiple recipes throughout the book.

Slow Cooker Tips

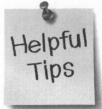

• All cooking times are a guide. Make sure you get to know your own slow cooker so that you can adjust timings accordingly.
• Read the manufacturers operating instructions as appliances can vary. For example, some recommend preheating the slow cooker for 20 minutes before use whilst others advocate switching on only when

you are ready to start cooking.
• Slow cookers do not brown-off meat. While not always necessary, if you do prefer to brown your meat you must first do this in a pan with a little low calorie cooking spray.
• A spray of one calorie cooking oil in the cooker before adding ingredients will help with cleaning or you can buy liners.
• Don't be tempted to regularly lift the lid of your appliance while cooking. The seal that is made with the lid on is all part of the slow cooking process. Each time you do lift the lid you will need to increase the cooking time.
• Removing the lid at the end of the cooking time can be useful to thicken up a sauce by adding additional cooking time and continuing to cook without the lid on. On the other hand if perhaps a sauce it too thick removing the lid and adding a little more liquid can help.
Always add hot liquids to your slow cooker, not cold.
• Do not overfill your slow cooker.
• Allow the inner dish of your slow cooker to completely cool before cleaning. Any stubborn marks can usually be removed after a period of soaking in hot soapy water.
• Be confident with your cooking. Feel free to use substitutes to suit your own taste and don't let a missing herb or spice stop you making a meal - you'll almost always be able to find something to replace it.

Our Recipes
The recipes in this book are all low calorie dishes mainly serving 4, which make it easier for you to monitor your overall daily calorie intake as well as those you are cooking for. The recommended daily calories are approximately 2000 for women and 2500 for men.

Broadly speaking, by consuming the recommended levels of calories each day you should maintain your current weight. Reducing the number of calories (a calorie deficit) will result in losing weight. This happens because the body begins to use fat stores for energy to make up the reduction in calories, which in turn results in weight loss. We have already counted the calories for each dish making it easy for you to fit this into your daily eating plan whether you want to lose weight, maintain your current figure or are just looking for some great-tasting, skinny slow cooker meals.

I'm Already On A Diet. Can I Use These Recipes?
Yes of course. All the recipes can be great accompaniments to many of the popular calorie-counting diets. We all know that sometimes dieting can result in hunger pangs, cravings and boredom from eating the same old foods day in and day out. Our skinny slow cooker recipes provide filling meals that should satisfy you for hours afterwards.
I Am Only Cooking For One. Will This Book Work For Me? Yes. We would recommend following the method for 4 servings then dividing and storing the rest in single size portions for you to use in the future. Most of the recipes will freeze well. Allow your slow cooked meals to cool to room temperature before refrigerating or freezing. When ready to defrost, allow to thaw in a fridge overnight then at room temperature for a few hours depending on the size of portion. Reheat thoroughly.

Nutrition
All of the recipes in this collection are balanced low calorie meals that should keep you feeling full and help

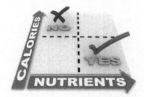

you avoid snacking in-between meals.

If you are following a diet, it is important to balance your food between proteins, good carbs, dairy, fruit and vegetables.

• **Protein.** Keeps you feeling full and is also essential for building body tissue. Good protein sources come from meat, fish and eggs.

• **Carbohydrates.** Carbs are generally high in calories, which make them difficult to include in a calorie limiting diet. Carbs are a good source of energy for your body as they are converted more easily into glucose (sugar), providing energy. Try to eat 'good carbs' which are high in fibre and nutrients e.g. whole fruits and veg, nuts, seeds, whole grain cereals, beans and legumes.

• **Dairy.** Dairy products provide you with vitamins and minerals. Cheeses can be high in calories but other products such as fat free Greek yoghurt, crème fraiche and skimmed milk are all good.

• **Fruit & Vegetables.** Eat your five a day. There is never a better time to fill your 5 a day quota. Not only are fruit and veg very healthy, they also fill up your plate and are ideal snacks when you are feeling hungry.

We have adopted the broader nutritional principals in all our recipes.

Portion Sizes
The majority of recipes are for 4 servings. The calorie count

is based on one serving. It is important to remember that if you are aiming to lose weight using any of our skinny

recipes, the size of the portion that you put on your plate will significantly affect your weight loss efforts. Filling your plate with over-sized portions will obviously increase your calorie intake and hamper your dieting efforts.
It is important with all meals that you use a correct sized portion, which generally is the size of your clenched fist. This applies to any side dishes of vegetables and carbs too.

All Recipes Are A Guide Only
All the recipes in this book are a guide only. You may need to alter quantities and cooking times to suit your own appliances.

THE

Skinny SLOW
COOKER
SUMMER
RECIPE BOOK

Summer Soups

Fresh Beetroot & Cream Soup
Serves 4

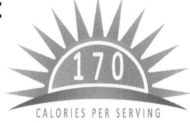

Ingredients:

2 onions, sliced
400g/14oz beetroot, cubed
150g/5oz potatoes, chopped
1lt/4 cups vegetable stock/ broth
2 tbsp freshly chopped basil
60ml/¼ cup single cream
Low cal cooking oil spray
Salt & pepper to taste

Method:

• Gently sauté the onion in a little low cal oil for a few minutes until softened.
• Add all the ingredients to the slow cooker, except the single cream.
• Combine well, cover and leave to cook on high for 1-2 hours or until the vegetables are cooked through.
• Place in a blender and blend to a smooth consistency.
• Check the seasoning, divide into bowls and pour a swirl of single cream into each bowl.

Beetroot is a beautiful much undervalued vegetable, which is the star of this recipe.

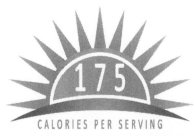

CALORIES PER SERVING

Parsnip & Sweet Apple Soup
Serves 4

Method:

- Gently sauté the onion & garlic in a little low cal oil for a few minutes until softened.
- Add all the ingredients to the slow cooker. Combine well, cover and leave to cook on high for 1-2 hours or until the parsnips are cooked through.
- Place in a blender and blend to a smooth consistency.
- Check the seasoning and serve.

Ingredients:

1 onion, sliced
1 garlic clove, crushed
300g/11oz parsnips, cubed
300g/11oz eating apples, peeled, cored & finely chopped
1lt/4 cups vegetable stock/broth
Low cal cooking oil spray
Salt & pepper to taste

Use sweet eating apples for this recipe rather than tart cooking apples.

17

Spring Pea & Parmesan Soup
Serves 4

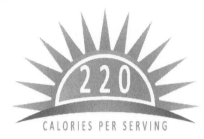

CALORIES PER SERVING

Ingredients:

2 onions, chopped
1 garlic clove, crushed
200g/7oz potatoes, chopped
400g/14oz fresh peas
750ml/3 cups vegetable stock/broth
250ml/1 cup semi skimmed/half fat milk
50g/2oz grated Parmesan cheese
3 tbsp freshly chopped mint
Salt & pepper to taste
Low cal cooking oil spray

Method:

• Gently sauté the onions & garlic in a little low cal oil for a few minutes until softened.
• Add the sautéed onions, chopped potatoes, peas, stock & milk to the slow cooker. Combine well, cover and leave to cook on high for 1-1½ hours or until the vegetables are tender.
• Place in a blender and blend to a smooth consistency.
• Season, sprinkle with grated Parmesan & chopped mint and serve.

Frozen peas are also fine to use for this recipe if you prefer but you will need to increase the cooking time by 30 mins.

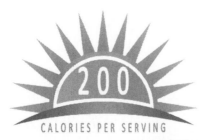

CALORIES PER SERVING

Summer Celery Soup

Serves 4

Method:

• Gently sauté the onion & celery in a little low cal oil for a few minutes until softened.

• Add all the ingredients to the slow cooker. Combine well, cover and leave to cook on high for 1-2 hours or until the sweet potatoes are tender.

• Place in a blender and blend to a smooth consistency, season and serve.

Ingredients:

1 onion, chopped
6 sticks celery, chopped
300g/11oz eating apples, peeled, cored & chopped
300g/11oz sweet potato, chopped
1lt/4 cups vegetable stock/broth
1 tsp brown sugar
Salt & pepper to taste
Low cal cooking oil spray

Celery is a delicate ingredient, which complements the sweetness of the apples & sweet potatoes.

19

Spring Vegetable Soup
Serves 4

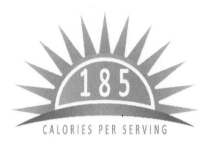

185

CALORIES PER SERVING

Ingredients:

2 leeks, chopped
2 garlic cloves, crushed
200g/7oz baby carrots, chopped
200g/7oz courgettes, chopped
200g/7oz potatoes, chopped
1 tsp dried mixed herbs
1lt/4 cups vegetable stock/ broth
Salt & pepper to taste
Low cal cooking oil spray

Method:

• Gently sauté the leek & garlic in a little low cal oil for a few minutes until softened.
• Add all the ingredients to the slow cooker. Combine well, cover and leave to cook on high for 1-2 hours or until the vegetables are all tender.
• Place in a blender and blend to a smooth consistency, season and serve.

You can use any combination of spring vegetables you prefer for this dish. You could also consider not blending the soup and leaving it chunky.

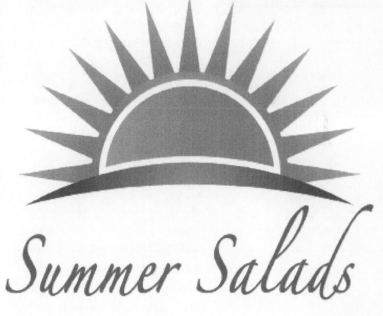

THE
Skinny SLOW
COOKER
SUMMER
RECIPE BOOK

Summer Salads

Glazed Beetroot & Rocket Citrus Salad

Serves 4

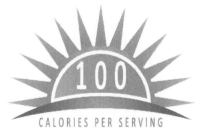

CALORIES PER SERVING

Ingredients:

6 beetroot bulbs

2 oranges

2 garlic cloves, crushed

1 onion, sliced

60ml/¼ cup balsamic vinegar

2 tbsp extra virgin olive oil

2 tbsp water

200g/7oz rocket

Salt & pepper to taste

Method:

• Give the beetroot bulbs a good scrub and cut each bulb into 6 even sized wedges. Grate the zest off one of the oranges and put to one side.

• Peel both the oranges and divide into segments.

• Place the beetroot wedges, orange segments, zest, garlic, sliced onion, balsamic vinegar, olive oil & water in the slow cooker. Combine well, cover and leave to cook on low for 3½-5 hours or until the beetroot wedges are tender.

• Allow to cool.

• Season and serve with the rocket, drizzling any leftover juices on to the top of the salad.

This delicious salad can be served warm or cold. Try adding a little goat's cheese and some freshly chopped flat leaf parsley when serving if you wish.

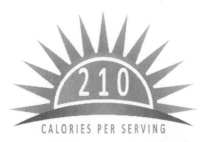

CALORIES PER SERVING

Greek Aubergine Salad
Serves 4

Method:

- Combine the aubergines, onions, dried spices, garlic, lemon juice & olive oil in the slow cooker. Cover and leave to cook on high for 2-3 hours or until the aubergine cubes are tender and still have their shape.
- Season and arrange on plates in the centre of the mixed leaves.
- Share the pitta bread fingers between the plates and add a dollop of Greek yoghurt to the side.
- Serve with the lemon wedges.

Ingredients:

3 aubergines, cut into 3cm cubes
1 onion, sliced
½ tsp each ground nutmeg & cinnamon
1 garlic clove, crushed
1 tbsp lemon juice
2 tbsp extra virgin olive oil
200g/7oz mixed leaves
2 regular pitta breads, cut into 3cm fingers
4 tbsp fat free Greek yoghurt
Lemon wedges to serve
Salt & pepper to taste

You could sprinkle a little paprika over the Greek yoghurt if you have it.

Spanish Chorizo Salad
Serves 4

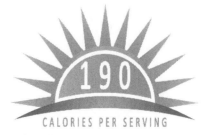

CALORIES PER SERVING

Ingredients:

150g/5oz chorizo sausage, diced
1 onion, sliced
1 red pepper, sliced
2 garlic cloves, crushed
400g/14oz vine ripened tomatoes, quartered
1 tbsp water
1 tsp brown sugar
Pinch of salt
200g/7oz mixed leaves
3 tbsp freshly chopped flat leaf parsley
Salt & pepper to taste

Method:

• Combine the diced chorizo, onion, peppers, garlic, tomatoes, water, sugar & salt in the slow cooker.
• Cover and leave to cook on high for 2-3 hours or until tender and cooked through.
• Season and arrange on plates with the mixed salad leaves.

This dish is also great served on top of low cal crispbreads or rice cakes.

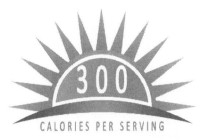

Beef & Chilli Salad

Serves 4

Method:

- Combine the steak, chillies, ginger, onions, peppers, garlic & stock in the slow cooker.
- Cover and leave to cook on low for 6-8 hours or until the beef is super tender (add a little more stock during cooking if needed).
- Season and arrange on plates with the baby leaf salad and chopped parsley.

Ingredients:

400g/14oz lean braising steak, cut into strips
2 red chillies, sliced
2 tsp freshly grated ginger
1 onion, sliced
1 red pepper, sliced
2 garlic cloves, finely sliced
250ml/1 cup beef stock/ broth
200g/7oz baby leaf salad
2 tbsp freshly chopped flat leaf parsley
Salt & pepper to taste

You could garnish with freshly chopped coriander to add a different twist to the salad.

Anchovy & Broccoli Salad
Serves 4

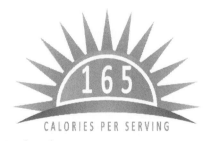

CALORIES PER SERVING

Ingredients:

400g/14oz tenderstem broccoli, roughly chopped
200g/7oz salad potatoes, sliced
6 tinned anchovy fillets, drained
½ tsp crushed chilli flakes
1 onion, sliced
2 garlic cloves, crushed
125ml/½ cup vegetable stock/broth
4 baby gem lettuces, shredded
Lemon wedges to serve
Salt & pepper to taste

Method:

• Combine all the ingredients, except the lettuce & lemon wedges, in the slow cooker.
• Cover and leave to cook on high for 2-4 hours or until the broccoli & potato slices are tender.
• Season and arrange on plates with the lettuce and lemon wedges.

You could also toss this dish through pasta to make a more substantial meal (leave out the lettuce).

Simple Shredded Chicken Salad
Serves 4

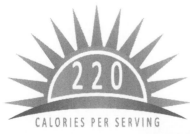

220
CALORIES PER SERVING

Method:

- Combine the chicken, garlic, stock, paprika & dried herbs in the slow cooker. Cover and leave to cook on high for 3-4 hours or until the chicken is super tender.
- Remove the chicken breasts and use two forks to shred.
- Serve with the fresh cherry tomatoes, shredded lettuce & chopped parsley.
- Drizzle some of the stock juices over the top of the salad if you wish.

Ingredients:

500g/1lb 2oz skinless chicken breasts
1 garlic clove, crushed
500ml/2 cups chicken stock/broth
½ tsp paprika
1 tsp mixed dried herbs
200g/7oz cherry tomatoes, halved
2 large romaine lettuces, shredded
2 tbsp freshly chopped flat leaf parsley
Salt & pepper to taste

This can be served hot or cold and is also great as a sandwich filling.

Pesto & Tomato Chicken Salad

Serves 4

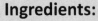

240

CALORIES PER SERVING

Ingredients:

500g/1lb 2oz skinless chicken breasts
200g/7oz cherry tomatoes, halved
2 tbsp green pesto
200g/7oz mixed baby leaf salad
2 tbsp freshly chopped flat leaf parsley
Salt & pepper to taste

Method:

• Combine the chicken, tomatoes, & pesto in the slow cooker. Cover and leave to cook on high for 3-4 hours or until the chicken is super tender (add a little water during cooking if needed).
• Remove the chicken breasts and use two forks to shred.
• Arrange the shredded chicken with the cooked cherry tomatoes on top of the mixed leaves.
• Sprinkle with chopped parsley & serve.

Shop-bought pesto is fine, or try making your own if you have a plentiful supply of fresh basil.

28

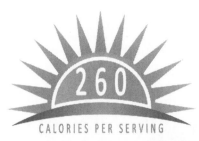

CALORIES PER SERVING

Coronation Salad
Serves 4

Method:

- Combine the chicken, onions, curry powder & stock in the slow cooker. Cover and leave to cook on high for 3-5 hours or until the chicken is super-tender.
- Remove the chicken breasts and use two forks to shred. Allow the chicken to cool. Combine with the yoghurt, mayonnaise & sultanas.
- Arrange on top of the rocket & spinach leaves.
- Sprinkle with chopped coriander & serve.

Ingredients:

500g/1lb 2oz skinless chicken breasts
1 onion, sliced
2 tbsp medium curry powder
60ml/¼ cup chicken stock/broth
1 tbsp fat free Greek yoghurt
1 tbsp low fat mayonnaise
1 tbsp sultanas, chopped
200g/7oz spinach & rocket leaves
1 tbsp freshly chopped coriander/cilantro
Salt & pepper to taste

You could garnish with some fresh red chilli slivers if you want an additional kick to this lovely dish.

Turkey Taco Salad
Serves 4

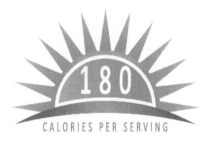

CALORIES PER SERVING

Ingredients:

350g/12oz lean turkey mince
200g/7oz ripe tomatoes, chopped
1 tbsp tomato puree/paste
1 onion, finely chopped
100g/3½oz sweetcorn
1 red pepper, chopped
2 tbsp taco seasoning
60ml/¼ cup chicken stock/broth
4 baby gem lettuces, shredded
2 tbsp fat free Greek yoghurt
1 tbsp freshly chopped flat leaf parsley
Salt & pepper to taste

Method:

• Combine the mince, tomatoes, puree, onions, sweetcorn, peppers, taco seasoning & stock in the slow cooker.
• Cover and leave to cook on high for 2-3 hours or low for 4-5 hours or until the mince is tender and cooked through.
• Arrange on top of the lettuce with a dollop of yoghurt, sprinkled with chopped parsley.

Use tinned chopped tomatoes if you don't have any fresh to hand.

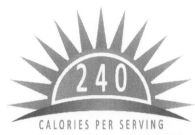

CALORIES PER SERVING

Honeyed Leek & Red Onion Pittas
Serves 4

Method:

- Add all the ingredients to the slow cooker, except the pitta bread, crème fraiche & cucumber batons.
- Combine well, cover and leave to cook on high for 2-4 hours or until the onions are soft & sweet.
- Serve in pitta pockets with the cucumber batons mixed inside & the crème fraiche on top.

Ingredients:

4 leeks, sliced
3 red onions, sliced
2 white onions, sliced
2 tbsp dried thyme
2 tbsp runny honey
60ml/¼ cup vegetable stock/broth
4 regular pitta bread
2 tbsp low fat crème fraiche
½ cucumber, cut into batons
Salt & pepper to taste

Any combination of onions will work fine for this recipe. If you have the time, sauté the onions & leek in a little low cal oil for a few minutes before adding to the slow cooker.

THE
Skinny SLOW
COOKER
SUMMER
RECIPE BOOK

Summer Pasta

Summer Squash & Chilli Linguine
Serves 4

310

Ingredients:

1 butternut squash, peeled, deseeded & cubed
1 onion, sliced
1 red chilli, sliced
1 garlic clove, crushed
120ml/½ cup vegetable stock/broth
2 tbsp low fat crème fraiche
300g/11oz linguine pasta
Low cal cooking oil spray
Salt & pepper to taste

Method:

• Add the squash, onion, chilli, garlic & vegetable stock to the slow cooker.
• Combine well, cover and leave to cook on low for 3-4 hours or until the squash is tender.
• Cook the linguine pasta in salted boiling water until tender.
• Take everything out of the slow cooker and place in a food processor.
• Add the crème fraiche and blitz until smooth.
• Toss with the drained linguine, season and serve.

Add a little more boiling water or stock if you feel the pasta sauce is a little thick when blending.

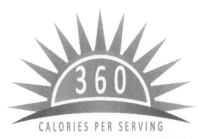

CALORIES PER SERVING

King Prawn Cherry Tomato Penne
Serves 4

Method:

- Add the onions, garlic, cherry tomatoes, tinned tomatoes, puree, stock cube & sugar to the slow cooker.
- Combine well, cover and leave to cook on low for 6-7 hours or until the sauce has thickened.
- Add the prawns and cook for a further hour or until the prawns are pink and cooked through.
- Meanwhile cook the penne pasta in salted boiling water until tender.
- Combine the cooked tomato sauce with the drained penne.
- Sprinkle with chopped basil and serve.

Ingredients:

1 onion, sliced
1 garlic clove, crushed
200g/7oz cherry tomatoes, halved
400g/14oz tinned chopped tomatoes
1 tbsp tomato puree/paste
½ vegetable stock cube, crumbled
½ tsp brown sugar
400g/14oz raw shelled king prawns
300g/11oz penne pasta
2 tbsp freshly chopped basil
Salt & pepper to taste

Use any type of pasta you prefer for this recipe.

Slow Cooked Spring Garlic Pasta
Serves 4

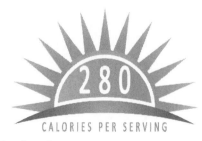

280
CALORIES PER SERVING

Ingredients:

1 whole head garlic
120ml/½ cup vegetable stock/broth
2 tbsp low fat crème fraiche
300g/11oz farfalle pasta
2 tbsp freshly chopped flat leaf parsley
Salt & pepper to taste

Method:

• Add the whole head of unpeeled garlic & stock to the slow cooker. Cover and leave to cook on low for 2-3 hours or until the garlic is soft.
• Meanwhile cook the farfalle pasta in salted boiling water until tender.
• Nip the tops of the garlic cloves with scissors and squeeze the softened garlic into a bowl.
• Combine with the crème fraiche and parsley.
• Toss with the drained pasta and serve.

Garlic is available all year round but locally sourced spring garlic is the sweetest of all. Serve with a simple green crunchy salad.

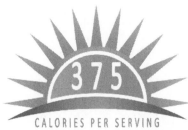

Lean Mini Meatballs & Fresh Herbs
Serves 4

Method:

- Place the turkey mince, garlic, breadcrumbs & fresh herbs in a food processor.
- Pulse for a few seconds to combine and use your hands to form the meat mixture into tiny meatballs about 2/3cm in diameter.
- Add meatballs, chopped tomatoes, puree and sugar to the slow cooker.
- Combine well, cover and leave to cook on low for 4-6 hours or until the meatballs are cooked through and the sauce is thickened.
- Meanwhile cook the spaghetti in salted boiling water until tender.
- Drain the pasta and divide into bowls.
- Load the meatballs and sauce on top and serve.

To make fresh breadcrumbs just put a slice of bread in the food processor and whizz for a few seconds.

Ingredients:

200g/7oz lean turkey mince
1 garlic clove
2 tbsp fresh breadcrumbs
2 tbsp mixed fresh herbs (basil, parsley & rosemary is a good mix)
400g/14oz tinned chopped tomatoes
2 tbsp tomato puree/paste
½ tsp brown sugar
300g/11oz spaghetti
Salt & pepper to taste

Vine Ripened Tomato Pasta Sauce
Serves 4

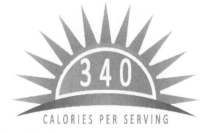

CALORIES PER SERVING

Ingredients:

800g/1¾lb vine ripened
tomatoes, quartered
2 tbsp balsamic vinegar
1 tbsp sundried tomato
puree/paste
2 tbsp water
1 tbsp olive oil
Pinch salt
1 garlic clove, crushed
300g/11oz tagliatelle
Salt & pepper to taste

Method:

• Place the tomatoes, balsamic vinegar, puree, water, oil, salt & garlic in the slow cooker.
• Combine well, cover and leave to cook on low for 3-5 hours or until tender.
• Meanwhile cook the tagliatelle in salted boiling water until tender.
• Toss the cooked tomatoes and juices through the drained pasta.
• Season and serve.

Fresh basil and Parmesan make lovely additional garnishes to this dish.

38

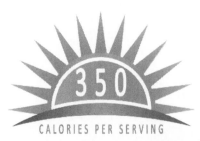

350 CALORIES PER SERVING

Pesto Prawn &Tenderstem Broccoli Spaghetti
Serves 4

Method:

- Place the broccoli, prawns, stock & pesto in the slow cooker. Combine well, cover and leave to cook on low for 3-4 hours or until the broccoli is tender and the prawns are cooked through.
- Meanwhile cook the spaghetti in salted boiling water until tender.
- Toss the cooked pesto prawns, broccoli and juices through the drained spaghetti.
- Season and serve with lemon wedges.

Ingredients:

200g/7oz tenderstem broccoli, roughly chopped
400g/14oz raw shelled king prawns
120ml/½ cup vegetable stock/broth
2 tbsp green pesto
300g/11oz spaghetti
Lemon wedges to serve
Salt & pepper to taste

You could also toss some fresh rocket leaves through the pasta just before serving.

Summer Vegetable Pasta
Serves 4

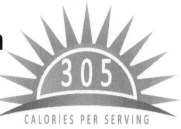

305
CALORIES PER SERVING

Ingredients:

400g/14oz courgettes,
mini corn & mushrooms
200g/7oz cherry tomatoes,
chopped
60ml/¼ cup vegetable
stock/broth
2 garlic cloves, crushed
2 tbsp tomato puree/paste
1 tbsp dried herbs
2 tbsp low fat crème
fraiche
300g/11oz conchiglie pasta
Salt & pepper to taste

Method:

• Slice the vegetables lengthways
into similar sizes and place in the
slow cooker along with the cherry
tomatoes, stock, garlic, puree & herbs.
• Combine well, cover and leave to
cook on low for 3-4 hours or until
tender.
• Meanwhile cook the pasta in salted
boiling water until tender.
• Stir the crème fraiche through the
cooked vegetables and toss with the
drained pasta.
• Season and serve.

*Chop the cherry tomatoes quite
finely to create a base for the
sauce.*

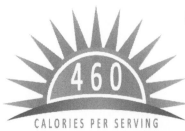

Chicken, Honey & Olive Pasta
Serves 4

Method:

- Place the chicken, honey, sliced lemon, stock, olives & garlic in the slow cooker. Combine well, cover and leave to cook on high for 3-4 hours or until the chicken is tender & cooked through.
- Use two forks to shred the chicken and return to the slow cooker.
- Meanwhile cook the pasta in salted boiling water until tender.
- Pick out the lemon slices & toss the chicken and olives through the pasta with the olive oil.
- Use any left over stock in the pot if you need to loosen it up.
- Sprinkle with chopped parsley, season & serve.

Ingredients:

400g/14oz skinless chicken breasts
2 tsp runny honey
½ lemon cut into thin slices
120ml/½ cup chicken stock/broth
100g/3½oz pitted olives, halved
1 garlic clove, crushed
1 tbsp olive oil
300g/11oz fusilli bucati pasta
2 tbsp freshly chopped parsley
Salt & pepper to taste

Bucati pasta is a twisted spaghetti-type pasta which holds oil & sauce really well, but any pasta will work fine.

41

Southern Italy's Summer Sauce
Serves 4

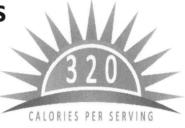

CALORIES PER SERVING

Ingredients:

300g/11oz fresh cherry tomatoes, halved
120ml/½ cup tomato passata/sieved tomatoes
2 garlic cloves, crushed
½ tsp brown sugar
1 tbsp capers, roughly chopped
6 tinned anchovy fillets, drained
25g/1oz sultana, roughly chopped
300g/11oz tagliolini pasta
2 tbsp freshly chopped basil
Salt & pepper to taste

Method:

• Place the cherry tomatoes, passata, garlic, sugar, capers, anchovies & sultanas in the slow cooker.
• Combine well, cover and leave to cook on high for 3-4 hours or until the tomatoes are very soft and the anchovy fillets are dissolved into the sauce.
• Meanwhile cook the pasta in salted boiling water until tender.
• Pour the sauce on top of the drained pasta, toss really well and sprinkle with chopped basil.

This dish is a real taste of rustic Southern Italy. Serve with a simple green & onion salad.

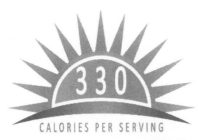

CALORIES PER SERVING

Pumpkin & Rosemary Riccioli

Serves 4

Method:

- Add the pumpkin, onion, chilli, garlic, vegetable stock, mustard & rosemary to the slow cooker. Combine well, cover and leave to cook on low for 3-4 hours or until the pumpkin is completely soft.
- Meanwhile cook the riccolio pasta in salted boiling water until tender.
- Take everything out of the slow cooker and place in a food processor.
- Add the olive oil and blitz until smooth, use a little boiling water to loosen the sauce if needed.
- Toss with the drained pasta, season and serve.

Ingredients:

1 medium pumpkin, peeled, deseeded & cubed
1 onion, sliced
½ red chilli, finely chopped
2 garlic cloves, crushed
120ml/½ cup vegetable stock/broth
1 tsp Dijon mustard
2 tsp freshly chopped or dried rosemary
1 tbsp olive oil
300g/11oz ricciloi pasta
Low cal cooking oil spray
Salt & pepper to taste

Ricciloi pasta is a spiral tube-type pasta great for smooth sauces, but you can use whichever pasta you have to hand.

Skinny SLOW COOKER SUMMER RECIPE BOOK

Summer Risotto

Pancetta Risotto
Serves 4

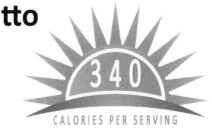

340

CALORIES PER SERVING

Ingredients:

75g/3oz pancetta bacon, trimmed & diced
1 onion, sliced
1 garlic clove, crushed
300g/11oz Arborio risotto rice
1lt/4 cups chicken stock/ broth
200g/7oz rocket
Low cal cooking oil spray
Salt & pepper to taste

Method:

• First sauté the pancetta, onion & garlic in a little low cal oil for a few minutes.
• Remove from the pan and chop as finely as possible. Return to the pan and add the rice. Stir around well to coat the rice in the residual oil.
• Place the contents of the pan in the slow cooker along with the stock. Combine well, cover and leave to cook on low for approx 2 hours or until the stock has been absorbed.
• Check the rice; if it is not tender add a some more stock and leave to cook for a little longer.
• When the risotto is tender and the stock has been absorbed, season and serve with the rocket.

Chopping the sautéed pancetta and onions as small as possible means their lovely salty sweet flavour will permeate every mouthful of this lovely risotto.

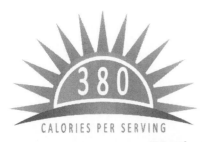

CALORIES PER SERVING

Spring Pea & Parmesan Risotto
Serves 4

Method:

- First sauté the onion & garlic in the olive oil for a few minutes.
- Add the rice to the pan and stir well to coat each grain in the olive oil.
- Place the contents of the pan in the slow cooker along with the stock and peas. Combine well, cover and leave to cook on low for approx 2 hours or until the stock has been absorbed.
- Check the rice; if it is not tender add a some more stock and leave to cook for a little longer.
- When the risotto is tender and the stock has been absorbed, season and serve with the Parmesan shavings on top.

Ingredients:

1 onion, sliced
2 garlic cloves, crushed
1 tbsp olive oil
300g/11oz Arborio risotto rice
1lt/4 cups chicken or vegetable stock/broth
300g/7oz fresh peas
25g/1oz Parmesan cheese shavings
Salt & pepper to taste

Frozen peas will work just as nicely as fresh peas. If you are using fresh peas you may wish hold off adding them the slow cooker until 30 minutes before the end of cooking so that they retain some 'crunch'.

Tomato & Fresh Basil Risotto
Serves 4

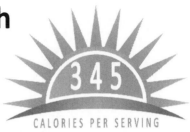

345 CALORIES PER SERVING

Ingredients:

1 onion, sliced
2 garlic cloves, crushed
1 tbsp olive oil
300g/11oz Arborio risotto rice
400g/14oz fresh chopped tomatoes
500ml/2 cups chicken or vegetable stock/broth
125g/4oz rocket
4 tbsp freshly chopped basil
Salt & pepper to taste

Method:

• First sauté the onion & garlic in the olive oil for a few minutes.
• Add the rice to the pan and stir well to coat each grain in the olive oil.
• Place the contents of the pan in the slow cooker along with the chopped tomatoes & stock. Combine well, cover and leave to cook on low for approx 2 hours or until all the liquid has been absorbed.
• Check the rice; if it is not tender add a some more stock and leave to cook for a little longer.
• When the risotto is tender and the stock has been absorbed, season and serve with the chopped basil on top and the rocket on the side.

You could also add a little sundried tomato paste to this dish to give additional depth.

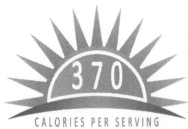

Butternut Squash& Goats Cheese Risotto
Serves 4

Method:

- First sauté the squash, onion & garlic in the olive oil for a few minutes (ensure you cut the squash finely otherwise you will find the rice is tender before the squash is ready).
- Add the rice to the pan and stir well to coat each grain in the olive oil.
- Place the contents of the pan in the slow cooker along with the stock. Combine well, cover and leave to cook on low for approx 2 hours or until all the liquid has been absorbed.
- Check the rice; if it is not tender add a some more stock and leave to cook for a little longer.
- When the risotto is tender and the stock has been absorbed, season and serve with the goat's cheese crumbled over the top.

Add a little dried sage to the slow cooker if you have it or garnish with fresh sage leaves if you like.

Ingredients:

1 large butternut squash, peeled, deseeded & sliced into matchsticks
1 onion, sliced
2 garlic cloves, crushed
1 tbsp olive oil
300g/11oz Arborio risotto rice
1lt/4 cups chicken or vegetable stock/broth
50g/2oz goat's cheese, crumbled
Salt & pepper to taste

Porcini Mushroom & Leek Risotto
Serves 4

330 CALORIES PER SERVING

Ingredients:

1 leek, sliced
75g/3oz porcini mushrooms, very finely chopped
2 garlic cloves, crushed
1 tbsp olive oil
300g/11oz Arborio risotto rice
1lt/4 cups chicken or vegetable stock/broth
200g/7oz crisp lettuce, shredded
Salt & pepper to taste

Method:

• First sauté the leek, mushrooms & garlic in the olive oil for a few minutes.
• Add the rice to the pan and stir well to coat each grain in the olive oil.
• Place the contents of the pan in the slow cooker along with the stock. Combine well, cover and leave to cook on low for approx 2 hours or until all the liquid has been absorbed.
• Check the rice; if it is not tender add a some more stock and leave to cook for a little longer.
• When the risotto is tender and the stock has been absorbed, season and serve with the shredded lettuce.

Grated Parmesan cheese is lovely sprinkled on almost any risotto but be sparing, as it will add to the calories of the dish.

THE
Skinny SLOW COOKER SUMMER
RECIPE BOOK

Summer Seafood

Fresh Mackerel & Summer Season Peppers
Serves 4

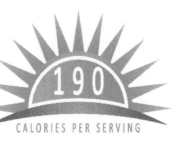

190

Ingredients:

2 yellow or orange peppers, sliced

2 onions, sliced

1 garlic clove, crushed

1 red chilli, finely sliced

250ml/1 cup fish stock

400g/14oz fresh whole mackerel, gutted

200g/7oz ripe plum tomatoes, chopped

2 tbsp tomato puree

200g/7oz rocket

Low cal cooking oil spray

Salt & pepper to taste

Method:

• Gently sauté the peppers, onions, garlic & chilli in a little low cal spray until softened.

• Add the sautéed vegetables to the slow cooker along with all the other ingredients, except the rocket.

• Gently combine, cover and leave to cook on low for 4-6 hours or until the fish is tender and cooked through.

• Gently lift out of the slow cooker (try to keep the fish whole), season and serve with the rocket leaves.

Use yellow or orange peppers rather than un-ripened green peppers.

52

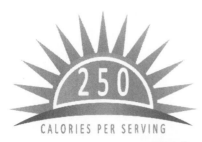

Fresh Herbed Salmon
Serves 4

Method:

- Place the salmon, stock and half the chopped herbs in the slow cooker. Gently combine, cover and leave to cook on high for 1-2 hours or until the fish is tender and cooked through.
- Mix the rest of the chopped herbs together with the mayonnaise, a squeeze of lemon and some salt & pepper.
- Remove the salmon fillets from the slow cooker.
- Spread the herbed mayonnaise onto the salmon fillets and serve with salad leaves and lemon wedges to serve.

Ingredients:

500g/1lb 2oz boneless salmon fillets
250ml/1 cup fish stock
4 tbsp freshly chopped flat leaf parsley
4 tbsp freshly chopped basil
3 tbsp low fat mayonnaise
Lemon wedges to serve
200g/7oz mixed green salad leaves
Low cal cooking oil spray
Salt & pepper to taste

You can alter the mix of fresh herbs to suit your own taste. Chives and coriander make a good alternative.

Caribbean Spiced Scallops
Serves 4

Ingredients:

2 red peppers, sliced
200g/7oz ripe plum tomatoes, roughly chopped
500g/1lb 2oz prepared fresh scallops
250ml/1 cup fish stock
½ tsp each ground all spice, chilli powder, coriander/cilantro & paprika
1 bunch spring onions/ scallions roughly chopped
2 large romaine lettuces, shredded
Low cal cooking oil spray
Salt & pepper to taste

Method:

• First gently sauté the peppers & plum tomatoes in a little low cal oil for a few minutes until softened.
• Place the scallops, stock, dried spices, spring onions, sautéed peppers & plum tomatoes in the slow cooker.
• Gently combine, cover and leave to cook on high for 45 minutes - 1 hour or until the scallops are cooked through.
• Gently lift the scallops, tomatoes & peppers out of the slow cooker.
• Season and serve with the shredded lettuce.

Sweet potato mash makes a great side to this Caribbean dish.

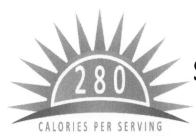

280

CALORIES PER SERVING

Lime Shrimps With Baby Spinach Leaves & Rice

Serves 4

Method:

- Place the prawns, coconut milk, lime juice, fish sauce, sugar, chilli & spinach in the slow cooker.
- Gently combine, cover and leave to cook on high for 45 minutes - 1 hour or until the prawns are cooked through.
- Meanwhile cook the rice in salted boiling water until tender.
- Serve the prawns and coconut milk on top of the drained rice with freshly chopped coriander sprinkled on top.

Ingredients:

500g/1lb 2oz raw shelled king prawns
250ml/1 cup low fat coconut milk
2 tbsp lime juice
1 tbsp Thai fish sauce
1 tsp brown sugar
1 red chilli, finely sliced
200g/7oz baby spinach leaves
4 tbsp freshly chopped coriander/cilantro
200g/7oz long grain rice
Low cal cooking oil spray
Salt & pepper to taste

Spinach is in season throughout late spring and summer. Baby leaves are the most sweet and tender.

Pineapple Curry King Prawns With Sugar Snap Peas

Serves 4

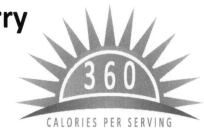

360 CALORIES PER SERVING

Ingredients:

1 onion, sliced
2 garlic cloves, crushed
500g/1lb 2oz raw shelled king prawns
250ml/1 cup low fat coconut milk
1 tbsp medium curry powder
1 tbsp lime juice
1 tbsp Thai fish sauce
2 tbsp tomato puree
200g/7oz fresh or tinned pineapple, roughly chopped
200g/7oz sugar snap peas
200g/7oz fine egg noodles
Low cal cooking oil spray
Salt & pepper to taste

Method:

• Gently sauté the onions & garlic in a little low cal oil for a few minutes until softened. Then place in the slow cooker.
• Add the prawns, coconut milk, curry powder, lime juice, fish sauce, tomato puree, pineapple & peas in the slow cooker.
• Gently combine, cover and leave to cook on high for 1-2 hours or until the prawns are cooked through.
• Meanwhile cook the noodles in salted boiling water until tender.
• Mix the drained noodles, prawns and sauce together & serve.

You could serve the sugar snaps peas roughly chopped and raw in this lovely summer noodle dish if you prefer.

56

THE

Skinny SLOW
COOKER
SUMMER
RECIPE BOOK

Summer BBQ

Sunny Honey Drumsticks
Serves 4

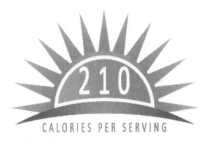

210

CALORIES PER SERVING

Ingredients:

8 skinless, chicken
drumsticks
1 tbsp runny honey
1 tbsp rice wine vinegar
3 garlic cloves, crushed
60ml/¼ cup soy sauce
1 tsp paprika
1 red onion, sliced
2 tbsp freshly chopped
parsley
Low cal cooking oil spray
Salt & pepper to taste

Method:

• First pierce the drumsticks with a
fork or skewer.
• Mix together the honey, rice wine
vinegar, garlic, soy sauce and paprika
to make a marinade. Smother the
drumsticks with this marinade and
leave to chill for as long as you can
(ideally overnight).
• After this time place the chicken
and juices in the slow cooker with a
little low cal spray. Cover and leave to
cook on high for 2-3 hours or until the
chicken is cooked through and piping
hot.
• Sprinkle with fresh parsley, season
and serve as part of a lovely summer
BBQ .

*Piercing the chicken will
encourage the marinade to
penetrate deep into the meat.*

58

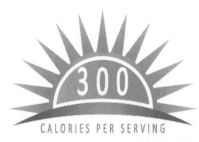

CALORIES PER SERVING

BBQ
Shredded Beef
Serves 4

Method:

- First place all the ingredients, except the stewing steak in a saucepan. Bring to the boil and reduce to a gentle simmer. Allow to cook for 8-10 minutes.
- Place in a blender and blitz into a smooth BBQ sauce.
- Check the seasoning and place the beef and BBQ sauce in the slow cooker. Cover and leave to cook on low for 8-10 hours or until the beef is meltingly tender (add a little water during cooking if you think the dish needs it).
- Remove from the slow cooker and use 2 forks to shred.
- Check the seasoning and serve.

Ingredients:

2 tbsp brown sugar
2 tbsp tomato puree/paste
2 onions, sliced
2 tbsp Dijon mustard
2 tbsp Worcestershire sauce
2 tbsp white wine vinegar
1 tsp paprika
3 garlic cloves crushed
120ml/½ cup tomato passata/paste
500g/1lb 2oz lean beef stewing steak, cubed
Salt & pepper to taste

This shredded BBQ beef is a perfect low maintenance addition to a family BBQ that you can prepare ahead of time.

Chicken & Pineapple Kebabs
Serves 4

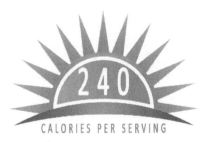

CALORIES PER SERVING

Ingredients:

500g/1lb 2oz skinless free range chicken, cubed
200g/7oz drained tinned pineapple chunks (reserve the juice)
2 red peppers, cut into chunks
2 tsp dried oregano
1 tsp garlic powder
8 skewers
Salt & pepper to taste

Method:

• Season the chicken and place in a bowl with the reserved pineapple juice and red peppers; combine well.
• Drain the juice from the bowl and sprinkle the chicken, pineapple & peppers with dried oregano & garlic powder.
• Skewer the chicken, pineapple & pepper pieces in turn and place in the slow cooker. Cover and leave to cook on high for 3-4 hours or until chicken is cooked through and tender.
• Check the seasoning and serve.

These light kebabs are delicious served with shredded salad and fat free Greek yoghurt for a perfect alfresco meal.

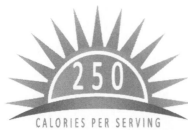

CALORIES PER SERVING

Sweet Sesame Salmon Kebabs
Serves 4

Method:

- Season and skewer the salmon pieces evenly.
- Mix together the sesame oil, soy sauce, honey, garlic & ginger and brush onto the salmon kebabs (reserving any leftover sauce).
- Cover and leave to cook on high for 1-2 hours or until the salmon is cooked through and tender.
- Brush with a little more sauce or water during cooking if the salmon is drying out.

Ingredients:

500g/1lb 2oz boneless
salmon fillets, cubed
1 tbsp sesame oil
2 tbsp soy sauce
1 tbsp runny honey
2 garlic cloves, crushed
½ tsp ground ginger
8 skewers
Salt & pepper to taste

You could add some baby sweetcorn or button mushrooms to these kebabs if you like.

Spiced Lamb Skewers
Serves 4

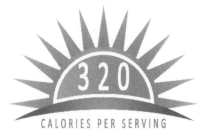

320

CALORIES PER SERVING

Ingredients:

500g/1lb 2oz lean lamb fillet

½ tsp each ground cumin, ginger & paprika

2 garlic cloves, crushed

12 cherry tomatoes

12 button mushrooms

2 tbsp freshly chopped coriander/cilantro

4 tbsp fat free Greek yoghurt

8 skewers

Low cal cooking oil spray

Salt & pepper to taste

Method:

• First brown the lamb in a frying pan on a high heat with a little low cal oil for a minute or two to seal the meat.
• Remove from the pan and place in a bowl with the whole tomatoes & mushrooms.
• Sprinkle the cumin, ginger, paprika & crushed garlic into the bowl and combine really well.
• Season and pierce the lamb, tomatoes and mushrooms in turn onto the skewers. Spray with a little oil and place in the slow cooker. Cover and leave to cook on high for 2-4 hours or until the lamb is cooked to your liking.
• Sprinkle with chopped coriander and serve with a dollop of Greek yoghurt for dipping.

Be sure not to overcook the lamb as you don't want it to be tough.

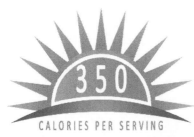

Sweet & Spicy Chicken Wings
Serves 4

Method:

- First pierce the wings with a fork or skewer.
- Mix together the honey, mustard, garlic & Worcestershire sauce and brush all over the wings.
- Place in the slow cooker with a little low cal spray, cover and leave to cook on high for 2-3 hours or until the chicken is cooked through and piping hot.
- Sprinkle with finely chopped spring onions and serve.

Ingredients:

15 skinless, chicken wings
2 tbsp runny honey
1 tsp English mustard
3 garlic cloves, crushed
3 tbsp Worcestershire sauce
A large bunch spring onions/scallions, finely chopped
Low cal cooking oil spray
Salt & pepper to taste

These wings are delicious served with homemade coleslaw, but be careful not to make it too calorific.

63

Tangy Apple Sauce
Serves 4

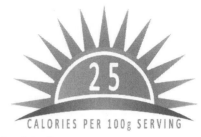

CALORIES PER 100g SERVING

Ingredients:

1kg/2¼lb cooking apples,
cored peeled & chopped
½ tsp ground cinnamon
500ml/2 cups water
3 tbsp brown sugar
Zest of 1 lemon

Method:

• Place the apples, cinnamon & water
in the slow cooker.
• Cover and leave to cook on low for
7-8 hours or until the apples are super
tender.
• Stir through the sugar & lemon
and cook for an hour longer. Chill and
serve.

*This is a lovely accompaniment
to BBQ cooked hot or cold
meats. You can serve chunky or
drain and whizz in a blender if
you prefer.*

64

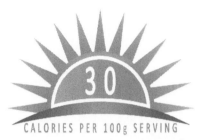

CALORIES PER 100g SERVING

Slow Cooked
Salsa
Serves 4

Method:

- Place the tomatoes, garlic, onion, cumin, ground coriander, chopped chillies, passata and sugar in the slow cooker. Cover and leave to cook on low for 4-5 hours or until the tomatoes have broken down and are super tender.
- Place in a food processor and pulse a few times.
- Stir through the reserved fresh onion to give the salsa a crunch and garnish with the freshly chopped coriander.
- Chill and serve.

Ingredients:

1kg/2¼lb ripe tomatoes, chopped
6 garlic cloves, crushed
2 onions, chopped (reserve 1 onion)
½ tsp each ground cumin & coriander/cilantro
2 red chillies, finely chopped
250ml/1 cup passata/ sieved tomatoes
1 tsp brown sugar
2 tbsp freshly chopped coriander/cilantro

Adjust the chilli to suit your own taste and serve as a fresh side to BBQ meats or with tortilla chips.

THE

Skinny SLOW
COOKER
SUMMER
RECIPE BOOK

Summer Vegetables

Summer Crustless Quiche

Serves 4

200 CALORIES PER SERVING

Ingredients:

200g/7oz cherry tomatoes, halved
1 red pepper, sliced
1 yellow pepper, sliced
125g/4oz courgettes, diced
125g/4oz aubergine/egg plant, diced
125g/4oz peas
2 garlic cloves, crushed
1 tsp dried mixed herbs
1 onion, sliced
6 free range eggs
200g/7oz rocket
Low cal cooking oil spray
Salt & pepper to taste

Method:

• Place the tomatoes, peppers, courgettes, aubergines, peas, garlic, herbs & sliced onions in the slow cooker. Spray well with a little low cal cooking oil. Combine, cover and leave to cook on high for 2 hours.
• Break the eggs into a bowl, gently whisk and pour into the slow cooker.
• Quickly combine for a few seconds. Replace the lid and leave to cook for a further 1-1½ hours or until the eggs are set and the vegetables are tender.
• Gently lift out of the slow cooker.
• Slice into thick wedges and serve with the rocket leaves.

This type of crust-less quiche is popular in Italy. Use whichever vegetables you have to hand to create your own version.

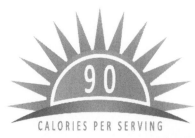

Portabella Mushrooms & Dolcelatte Cheese
Serves 4

Method:

- Place the mushrooms, garlic, stock & lemon juice in the slow cooker.
- Combine, cover and leave to cook on high for 2-4 hours or until most of the liquid has disappeared.
- Stir in the dolcelatte cheese and fresh basil.
- Check the seasoning and serve.

Ingredients:

600g/1lb 5oz portabella mushrooms, thickly sliced
2 garlic cloves, crushed
60ml/¼ cup vegetable stock/broth
1 tbsp lemon juice
50g/2oz dolcelatte cheese
2 tbsp freshly chopped basil
Low cal cooking oil spray
Salt & pepper to taste

These delicious mushrooms can be served as a luxurious side dish, on top of French toast or tossed through long cut spaghetti.

Sugar Snap & Aubergine Ratatouille

Serves 4

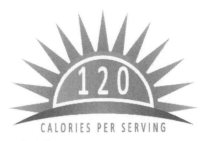

CALORIES PER SERVING

Ingredients:

200g/7oz sugar snap peas
200g/7oz baby courgettes, sliced lengthways
200g/7oz baby sweetcorn, sliced lengthways
1 aubergine, diced
2 yellow peppers, sliced
2 garlic cloves, crushed
1 vegetable stock cube, crumbled
800g/1¾lb tinned chopped tomatoes
1 tbsp tomato puree/paste
2 tbsp each freshly chopped basil & flat leaf parsley
Salt & pepper to taste

Method:

• Place all the ingredients in the slow cooker.
• Cover and leave to cook on high for 3-4 hours / low for 6-8 hours, or until the vegetables are tender.
• Check the seasoning and serve.

Of course you could also use fresh tomatoes rather than chopped tomatoes if you have enough to hand.

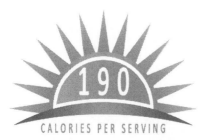

Paprika Sweet Potatoes
Serves 4

Method:

- Place all the ingredients in the slow cooker.
- Cover and leave to cook on high for 3-4 hours or until the sweet potatoes are tender but not falling apart.
- Check the seasoning and serve.

Ingredients:

500g/1lb 2oz sweet potatoes, cut into 4cm cubes
1 tsp paprika
1 red chilli, finely chopped
1 red onion, sliced
2 yellow peppers, sliced
2 garlic cloves, crushed
1 vegetable stock cube, crumbled
250ml/1 cup tomato passata/sieved tomatoes
400g/14oz tinned chopped tomatoes
½ tsp brown sugar
1 tbsp tomato puree/paste
Salt & pepper to taste

The sugar and seasoning will balance the acidity of the tomatoes, add a little more if needed.

71

Tender Leaf Spinach & Spiced Chickpeas

Serves 4

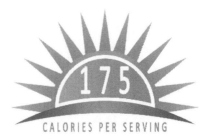

Ingredients:

300g/11oz baby spinach
leaves
400g/14oz tinned
chickpeas, drained
400g/14oz fresh ripe
tomatoes, roughly
chopped
1 onion, sliced
2 garlic cloves, crushed
1 tbsp medium or hot
curry powder
60ml/¼ cup vegetable
stock/broth
4 tbsp fat free Greek
yoghurt
Salt & pepper to taste

Method:

• Place all the ingredients, except the Greek yoghurt, in the slow cooker.
• Cover and leave to cook on low for 3-4 hours (add a little more stock during cooking if needed).
• Check the seasoning and serve with a dollop of Greek yoghurt on the side.

Add some chopped red chillies to garnish this dish if you like.

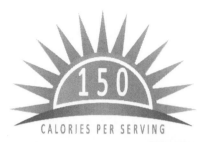

CALORIES PER SERVING

Slow Cooked Summer Peppers
Serves 4

Method:

• Place all the ingredients in the slow cooker. Cover and leave to cook on low for 6-8 (add a splash of water during cooking if needed).
• Check the seasoning and serve.
• If you love garlic you can squeeze the garlic pulp out of the cloves and mix with the peppers too.

Ingredients:

8 red, yellow or orange peppers, quartered
200g/7oz vine ripened tomatoes, halved
8 unpeeled garlic cloves
2 tsp brown sugar
2 tbsp olive oil
Salt & pepper to taste

Don't use green peppers as they can have a bitter taste which doesn't complement this recipe. Eat these slow cooked peppers just as they are or serve with salad, boiled rice or green salad.

73

Mozzarella & Basil Tomatoes
Serves 4

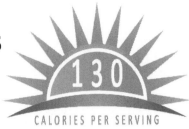

CALORIES PER SERVING

Ingredients:

1 tbsp olive oil
2 garlic cloves, crushed
1 tsp brown sugar
2 tsp balsamic vinegar
8 large beef tomatoes
3 tbsp water
100g/3½oz low fat
mozzarella cheese, roughly
chopped
3 tbsp freshly chopped
basil
Salt & pepper to taste

Method:

• Mix the oil, garlic, sugar & balsamic vinegar together.
• Halve the tomatoes and brush with the sweet garlic oil.
• Place in the slow cooker, with the water, cover and leave to cook on low for 4-6 hours (add a little more water during cooking if needed).
• When the tomatoes are tender sprinkle each on top with mozzarella cheese and continue cooking until the cheese melts.
• Remove from the slow cooker, sprinkle with basil and serve.

Cook the tomatoes long enough for them to be super-tender but not so that they lose their form and fall apart.

74

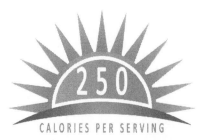

Smoky Pinto Beans & Fresh Spring Onions
Serves 4

Method:

- Slice the spring onions diagonally, mix with the chopped parsley and put to one side.
- Add the drained pinto beans, puree, sugar, peppers, stock, paprika & garlic to the slow cooker. Cover and leave to cook on high for 2-4 hours or until the stock has reduced and the smoky beans are tender.
- Remove from the slow cooker and divide into bowls.
- Check the seasoning, sprinkle with the fresh parsley & spring onion mix and serve.

Ingredients:

1 large bunch spring onions
3 tbsp freshly chopped flat leaf parsley
800g/1¾lb tinned pinto beans, drained & rinsed
1 tbsp tomato puree/paste
1 tsp brown sugar
200g/7oz shop bought roasted peppers, roughly chopped
120ml/½ cup vegetable stock/broth
1 tbsp smoked paprika
1 garlic clove, crushed
Salt & pepper to taste

Pinto beans are a staple of Mexican cooking. Garnishing with fresh spring onions gives this dish a light crunchy bite.

Cajun Spring Greens

Serves 4

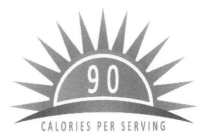

CALORIES PER SERVING

Ingredients:

500g/1lb 2oz shredded
spring greens
250ml/1 cup vegetable
stock/broth
1 tbsp Cajun seasoning
(or make your own by
mixing ½ tsp each paprika,
cayenne pepper, sea salt,
black pepper, cumin &
ground garlic)
1 garlic clove, crushed
Lemon wedges to serve
Salt & pepper to taste

Method:

• Add the spring greens, stock, Cajun seasoning & garlic to the slow cooker.
• Cover and leave to cook on high for 2-4 hours or until the stock has reduced and the spring greens are tender.
• Remove from the slow cooker, check the seasoning and serve with lemon wedges.

Handy bags of prepared shredded spring greens are readily available in most supermarkets.

76

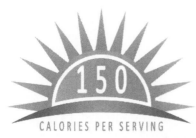

CALORIES PER SERVING

Sunshine Sweet Roasted Vegetables
Serves 4

Method:

- Add all the ingredients to the slow cooker and combine really well to make sure all the vegetables are properly coated.
- Cover and leave to cook on low for 4-6 hours or until all the vegetables are tender (add a splash of water during cooking if needed).
- Remove from the slow cooker, check the seasoning and serve.

Ingredients:

200g/7oz carrots, thickly sliced
200g/7oz sweet potatoes, thickly sliced
200g/7oz parsnips, thickly sliced
200g/7oz cherry tomatoes, halved
200g/7oz baby sweetcorn, sliced lengthways
1 red pepper, sliced
1 red onion, quartered and divided into segments
1 tbsp runny honey
1 tbsp balsamic vinegar
1 tbsp olive oil
1 tbsp water
1 tsp dried basil or mixed herbs
Salt & pepper to taste

This colourful roasted vegetable medley is a meal on its own or you could serve with a mixed salad.

THE Skinny SLOW COOKER SUMMER RECIPE BOOK

Summer Casseroles

Apricot & Pork Tenderloin Casserole
Serves 4

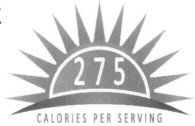

275
CALORIES PER SERVING

Ingredients:

2 yellow or orange
peppers, sliced
2 onions, sliced
1 garlic clove, crushed
500g/1lb 2oz pork
tenderloin, cut into 2cm
thick slices
125g/4oz dried apricots,
chopped
1 tsp brown sugar
200g/7oz ripe plum
tomatoes, chopped
2 tbsp tomato puree
Low cal cooking oil spray
Salt & pepper to taste

Method:

• Gently sauté the peppers, onions
& garlic in a little low cal spray until
softened.
• Add the sautéed vegetables to the
slow cooker along with all the other
ingredients.
• Gently combine, cover and leave to
cook on low for 3-5 hours or until the
pork is tender and cooked through.
• Season and serve.

*This dish is great served with
salad, flat bread or couscous.*

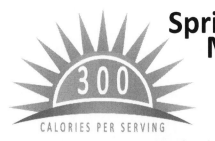

Spring Portabella Mushrooms & Chilli Steak Casserole
Serves 4

Method:

- Gently sauté the peppers, onions, garlic & mushrooms in a little low cal spray until softened.
- Add the sautéed vegetables to the slow cooker along with all the other ingredients, except the spring onions.
- Gently combine, cover and leave to cook on low for 7-9 hours or until the beef is meltingly tender (add a little more stock during cooking if needed).
- Season and serve with the sliced spring onions on top.

Ingredients:

2 red peppers, thinly sliced
2 onions, sliced
2 garlic cloves, finely sliced
4 large portabella mushrooms
500g/1lb 2oz lean beef stewing steak
2 tbsp soy sauce
2 tbsp Worcestershire sauce
60ml/¼ cup beef stock/broth
1 bunch spring onions/scallions, sliced lengthways into ribbons
Low cal cooking oil spray
Salt & pepper to taste

Large flat Portabella mushrooms are available all year round but they are at their best in the spring.

Marmalade Chicken Casserole
Serves 4

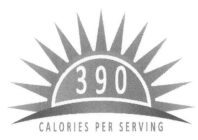

Ingredients:

500g/1lb 2oz skinless chicken breasts
1 tbsp plain/all purpose flour
2 garlic cloves, crushed
2 tbsp orange marmalade
60ml/¼ cup fresh orange juice
60ml/¼ cup chicken stock/broth
2 tbsp tomato puree/paste
½ tsp each brown sugar & salt
200g/7oz long grain rice
1 bunch spring onions/scallions, sliced lengthways into ribbons
Low cal cooking oil spray
Salt & pepper to taste

Method:

• First dust the chicken breast with flour until well covered and place in the slow cooker.
• Mix together the garlic, marmalade, orange juice, stock, puree, salt & sugar and add to the slow cooker covering the dusted chicken as much as possible. Cover and leave to cook on low for 4-5 hours or until the chicken is cooked through.
• Meanwhile cook the rice in salted boiling water until tender.
• Season and serve with the sliced spring onions and any juices drizzled over the top on a bed of boiled rice.

This is a light, sweet, summer supper, which the whole family will enjoy.

Fresh Ginger Cashew Chicken
Serves 4

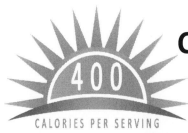

CALORIES PER SERVING

Method:

- First dust the cubed chicken with flour until well covered.
- Quickly brown the chicken in a frying pan with a little low cal oil.
- Place in the slow cooker with all the other ingredients, except the nuts & noodles. Cover and leave to cook on low for 3-4 hours or until the chicken is cooked through.
- Meanwhile cook the noodles in salted boiling water until tender.
- Toss the chicken, juices and noodles together and sprinkle the cashew nuts over the top.
- Season & serve.

Ingredients:

500g/1lb 2oz skinless chicken breasts, cubed
1 tbsp plain/all purpose flour
2 tbsp freshly grated ginger
2 garlic cloves, crushed
60ml/¼ chicken stock/broth
1 tbsp tomato puree/paste
½ tsp each brown sugar, crushed chilli flakes & salt
100g/3½oz cashew nuts
200g/7oz egg noodles
Low cal cooking oil spray
Salt & pepper to taste

Adding the cashew nuts as a garnish gives this dish a crunch. You can add them during cooking if your prefer.

White Bean & Summer Leek Chicken Stew
Serves 4

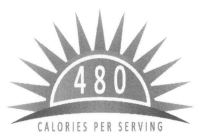

Ingredients:

2 leeks, chopped
2 garlic cloves, crushed
500g/1lb 2oz skinless
chicken breasts, cubed
60ml/¼ chicken stock/
broth
2 tsp dried rosemary
400g/14oz tinned white
beans, drained
200g/7oz egg noodles
Lime wedges to serve
1 avocado, diced
Low cal cooking oil spray
Salt & pepper to taste

Method:

• Gently sauté the leeks & garlic in a little low cal oil for a few minutes until softened.
• Place in the slow cooker with all the other ingredients, except the noodles, lime wedges & avocado. Cover and leave to cook on low for 3-4 hours or until the chicken is cooked through.
• Meanwhile cook the noodles in salted boiling water until tender.
• Toss the chicken stew and noodles together.
• Serve with the lime wedges on the side & diced avocado arranged over the top.

Adding the avocado & lime wedges give this dish a really fresh feel.

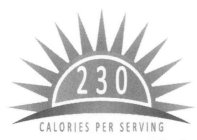

CALORIES PER SERVING

Fresh Basil & Parmesan Chicken Stew

Serves 4

Method:

- Gently sauté the onion & garlic in a little low cal oil for a few minutes until softened.
- Place in the slow cooker with all the other ingredients, except the Parmesan cheese. (Reserve a little fresh basil for garnish). Cover and leave to cook on low for 3-4 hours or until the chicken is cooked through.
- Season and serve.

Ingredients:

2 onions, sliced
2 garlic cloves, crushed
500g/1lb 2oz skinless chicken breasts, cubed
60ml/¼ cup chicken stock/broth
400g/14oz fresh ripe plum tomatoes
200g/7oz baby courgettes, sliced lengthways
50g/2oz Parmesan cheese
1 large bunch fresh basil, roughly chopped
Low cal cooking oil spray
Salt & pepper to taste

Feel free to use tinned tomatoes if you don't have fresh tomatoes to hand.

Chinese Beef & Pak Choi Casserole
Serves 4

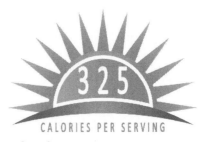

CALORIES PER SERVING

Ingredients:

500g/1lb 2oz lean beef stewing steak, cubed
1 tbsp plain/all purpose flour
1 tsp Chinese 5 spice powder
2 onions, sliced
4 garlic cloves, crushed
1 red chilli, finely chopped
250ml/1 cup beef stock/broth
3 pak choi sliced lengthways
3 tbsp soy sauce
1 tsp brown sugar
Low cal cooking oil spray
Salt & pepper to taste

Method:

• First toss the steak, flour and Chinese 5 spice together to cover the meat.
• Quickly brown in a frying pan with a little low cal spray and set to one side.
• Use the same pan to gently sauté the onions, garlic & chilli and then place everything in the slow cooker.
• Cover and leave to cook on low for 6-8 hours or until the beef is really tender (add a little more stock if needed during cooking).
• Season and serve.

Pak choi is a popular Chinese cabbage also known as bok choi. If you want it to retain some fresh crunch, hold off placing in the slow cooker until half an hour before the end of cooking.

86

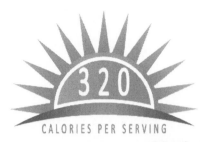

320
CALORIES PER SERVING

Celeriac & Orange Beef Stew
Serves 4

Method:

- Gently sauté the leeks & garlic until softened.
- Place everything in the slow cooker, except the baby sweetcorn, Cover and leave to cook on low for 6-8 hours or until the beef is really tender.
- 20 minutes before the end of cooking add the baby sweetcorn.
- Season and serve.

Ingredients:

2 leeks, sliced
3 garlic cloves, crushed
500g/1lb 2oz lean beef stewing steak, cubed
750g/1lb 11oz celeriac, diced
250ml/1 cup beef stock/ broth
60ml/ ¼ cup dry white wine
Juice and zest of 1 large orange
3 tbsp soy sauce
200g/7oz baby sweetcorn, chopped
Low cal cooking oil spray
Salt & pepper to taste

Beef stews can be quite heavy but this light stew is lifted by the citrus of the orange.

87

THE Skinny SLOW COOKER SUMMER RECIPE BOOK

Summer Fruit

Fresh Cherry & Almonds
Serves 4

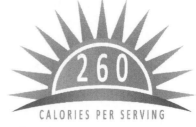

CALORIES PER SERVING

Ingredients:

800g/1¾lb cherries, deseeded
100g/3½oz brown sugar
60ml/¼ cup boiling water
3 tbsp chopped almonds
½ tsp vanilla extract

Method:

• Place all the ingredients in the slow cooker. Cover and leave to cook on high for 1-2 hours or until the cherries are tender and syrupy.
• Allow to cool and serve (sprinkle with a little more brown sugar if needed).

June is a wonderful month for fresh cherries. This dish is lovely served with low fat crème fraiche.

Poached August Pears

Serves 4

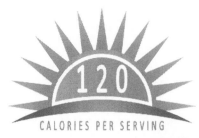

Method:

- Peel, core and halve the pears. Place all the ingredients in the slow cooker.
- Combine well, cover and leave to cook on high for 1-2 hours or until the pears are tender.
- Serve whilst warm with the juice spooned over the top.

Ingredients:

4 ripe pears
250ml/1 cup fresh orange juice
75g/3oz brown sugar
60ml/¼ cup boiling water
½ tsp vanilla extract

August is the first month domestic pears really come into season. Use the ripest pears you can get your hands on & serve with fat free Greek yoghurt if you like.

Fresh Cinnamon Stewed Apricots

Serves 4

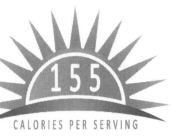

CALORIES PER SERVING

Ingredients:

12 ripe apricots, stoned & halved
250ml/1 cup water
125g/4oz brown sugar (reserve ½ tsp of sugar)
½ tsp vanilla extract
½ tsp ground cinnamon

Method:

• Stone and halve the fresh apricots. Place all the ingredients in the slow cooker.
• Combine well, cover and leave to cook on low for 4-6 hours or until the apricots are tender.
• Sprinkle with the reserved brown sugar and serve.

Late summer is the best month for domestic apricots. Enjoy these just as they are or with a little fresh ice cream.

92

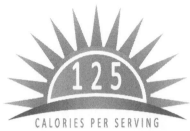

CALORIES PER SERVING

New Season Poached Strawberries
Serves 4

Method:

- Place all the ingredients in the slow cooker.
- Combine well, cover and leave to cook on high for 1-2 hours or until the strawberries are tender but not falling apart.
- Check the balance of the sweetness and serve.

Ingredients:

800g/1¾lb hulled ripe strawberries
75g/3oz brown sugar
60ml/¼ cup water
2 tbsp lemon juice

The first strawberries of the year are a welcome sight. Their natural sweetness is far superior to the 'forced' fruit that is available all year round.

Late Summer Plums
Serves 4

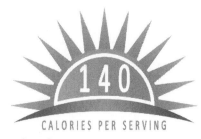

CALORIES PER SERVING

Ingredients:

800g/1¾lb plums, halved & deseeded
75g/3oz brown sugar
1 tbsp runny honey
2 tsp balsamic vinegar
250ml/1 cup boiling water
1 tbsp lemon juice

Method:

• Place all the ingredients in the slow cooker.
• Combine well, cover and leave to cook on high for 2-3 hours or until the plums are tender.
• Spoon the plums out of the slow cooker along with as much syrup as you wish.
• Check the balance of the sweetness and serve.

Late summer is when plums are harvested. Don't worry if they are not very ripe, this recipe will work well anyway.

94

Conversion Chart
Weights for dry ingredients:

Metric	Imperial
7g	¼ oz
15g	½ oz
20g	¾ oz
25g	1 oz
40g	1½oz
50g	2oz
60g	2½oz
75g	3oz
100g	3½oz
125g	4oz
140g	4½oz
150g	5oz
165g	5½oz
175g	6oz
200g	7oz
225g	8oz
250g	9oz
275g	10oz
300g	11oz
350g	12oz
375g	13oz
400g	14oz
425g	15oz
450g	1lb
500g	1lb 2oz
550g	1¼lb
600g	1lb 5oz
650g	1lb 7oz
675g	1½lb
700g	1lb 9oz
750g	1lb 11oz
800g	1¾lb
900g	2lb
1kg	2¼lb
1.1kg	2½lb
1.25kg	2¾lb
1.35kg	3lb
1.5kg	3lb 6oz
1.8kg	4lb
2kg	4½lb
2.25kg	5lb
2.5kg	5½lb
2.75kg	6lb

Conversion Chart

Liquid measures:

Metric	Imperial	Aus	US
25ml	1fl oz		
60ml	2fl oz	¼ cup	¼ cup
75ml	3fl oz		
100ml	3½fl oz		
120ml	4fl oz	½ cup	½ cup
150ml	5fl oz		
175ml	6fl oz	¾ cup	¾ cup
200ml	7fl oz		
250ml	8fl oz	1 cup	1 cup
300ml	10fl oz/½ pt	1¼ cups	
360ml	12fl oz		
400ml	14fl oz		
450ml	15fl oz	2 cups	2 cups/1 pint
600ml	1 pint	1 pint	2½ cups
750ml	1¼ pint		
900ml	1½ pints		
1 litre	1½ pints	1¾ pints	1 quart

CookNation

Other CookNation Titles

You may also be interested in other titles in the CookNation series. In particular, our popular series of slow cooker titles:

The Skinny Slow Cooker Recipe Book *#1 Amazon Best Seller*
More Skinny Slow Cooker Recipes *#1 Amazon Best Seller*
The Skinny Slow Cooker Soup Recipe Book
The Skinny Slow Cooker Vegetarian Recipe Book
The Skinny Slow Cooker Curry Recipe Book *#1 Amazon Best Seller*
The Skinny 5:2 Slow Cooker Recipe Book *#1 Amazon Best Seller*
The Paleo Diet For Beginners Slow Cooker Recipe Book

You can find all the following great titles by searching under '**CookNation**' on Amazon.

Review

If you enjoyed 'The Skinny Slow Cooker Summer Recipe Book' we'd really appreciate your feedback. Reviews help others decide if this is the right book for them so a moment of your time would be appreciated. Thank you.

The Skinny Slow Cooker Soup Recipe Book

Simple, Healthy & Delicious Low Calorie Soup Recipes For Your Slow Cooker. All Under 100, 200 & 300 Calories.
Paperback / Kindle

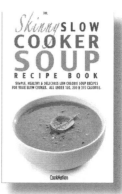

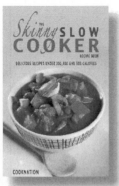

The Skinny Slow Cooker Recipe Book
40 Delicious Recipes Under 300, 400 And 500 Calories.

Paperback / Kindle

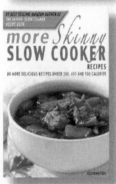

More Skinny Slow Cooker Recipes
75 More Delicious Recipes Under 300, 400 & 500 Calories.

Paperback / Kindle

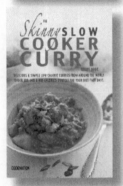

The Skinny Slow Cooker Curry Recipe Book
Delicious & Simple Low Calorie Curries From Around The World Under Under 200, 300 & 400 Calories. Perfect For Your Fast Days.

Paperback / Kindle

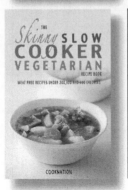

The Skinny Slow Cooker Vegetarian Recipe Book
40 Delicious Recipes Under 200, 300 And 400 Calories.

Paperback / Kindle

The Skinny 5:2 Slow Cooker Recipe Book

Skinny Slow Cooker Recipe And Menu Ideas Under 100, 200, 300 & 400 Calories For Your 5:2 Diet.

Paperback / Kindle

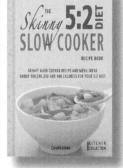

The Skinny 5:2 Curry Recipe Book

Spice Up Your Fast Days With Simple Low Calorie Curries, Snacks, Soups, Salads & Sides Under 200, 300 & 400 Calories

Paperback / Kindle

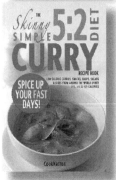

The Skinny Halogen Oven Family Favourites Recipe Book

Healthy, Low Calorie Family Meal-Time Halogen Oven Recipes Under 300, 400 and 500 Calories

Paperback / Kindle

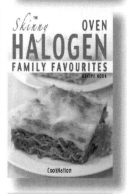

Skinny Halogen Oven Cooking For One

Single Serving, Healthy, Low Calorie Halogen Oven Recipes Under 200, 300 and 400 Calories

Paperback / Kindle

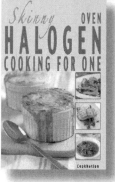

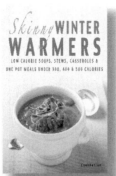

Skinny Winter Warmers Recipe Book

Soups, Stews, Casseroles & One Pot Meals Under 300, 400 & 500 Calories.

Paperback / Kindle

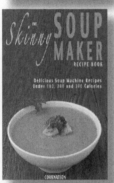

The Skinny Soup Maker Recipe Book

Delicious Low Calorie, Healthy and Simple Soup Recipes Under 100, 200 and 300 Calories. Perfect For Any Diet and Weight Loss Plan.
Paperback / Kindle

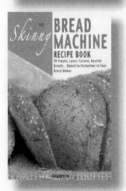

The Skinny Bread Machine Recipe Book

70 Simple, Lower Calorie, Healthy Breads...Baked To Perfection In Your Bread Maker.

Paperback / Kindle

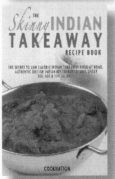

The Skinny Indian Takeaway Recipe Book

Authentic British Indian Restaurant Dishes Under 300, 400 And 500 Calories. The Secret To Low Calorie Indian Takeaway Food At Home

Paperback / Kindle

The Skinny Juice Diet Recipe Book

5lbs, 5 Days. The Ultimate Kick-Start Diet and Detox Plan to Lose Weight & Feel Great!

Paperback / Kindle

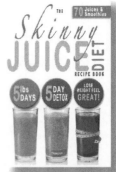

The Skinny 5:2 Diet Recipe Book Collection

All The 5:2 Fast Diet Recipes You'll Ever Need. All Under 100, 200, 300, 400 And 500 Calories

Kindle

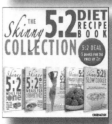

Available only on Kindle

The Skinny 5:2 Fast Diet Meals For One

Single Serving Fast Day Recipes & Snacks Under 100, 200 & 300 Calories

Paperback / Kindle

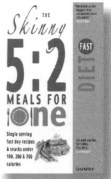

The Skinny 5:2 Fast Diet Vegetarian Meals For One

Single Serving Fast Day Recipes & Snacks Under 100, 200 & 300 Calories

Paperback / Kindle

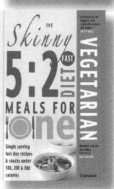

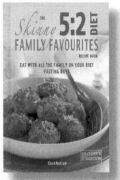

The Skinny 5:2 Fast Diet Family Favourites Recipe Book

Eat With All The Family On Your Diet Fasting Days

Paperback / Kindle

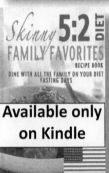

Available only on Kindle

The Skinny 5:2 Fast Diet Family Favorites Recipe Book *U.S.A. EDITION*

Dine With All The Family On Your Diet Fasting Days

Paperback / Kindle

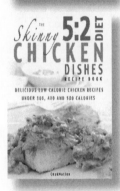

The Skinny 5:2 Diet Chicken Dishes Recipe Book

Delicious Low Calorie Chicken Dishes Under 300, 400 & 500 Calories

Paperback / Kindle

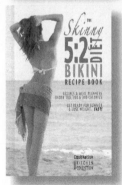

The Skinny 5:2 Bikini Diet Recipe Book

Recipes & Meal Planners Under 100, 200 & 300 Calories. Get Ready For Summer & Lose Weight...FAST!

Paperback / Kindle

The Paleo Diet For Beginners Slow Cooker Recipe Book

Gluten Free, Everyday Essential Slow Cooker Paleo Recipes For Beginners

Kindle

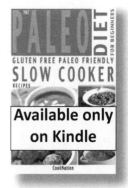

The Paleo Diet For Beginners Meals For One

The Ultimate Paleo Single Serving Cookbook

Paperback / Kindle

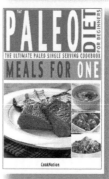

The Paleo Diet For Beginners Holidays

Thanksgiving, Christmas & New Year Paleo Friendly Recipes

Kindle

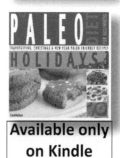

The Healthy Kids Smoothie Book

40 Delicious Goodness In A Glass Recipes for Happy Kids.

Kindle

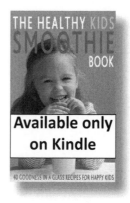

16550422R00059

Printed in Great Britain
by Amazon